Mediterranean Sea Cookbook

An Original Mediterranean Cooking Plan

Joseph Bellisario

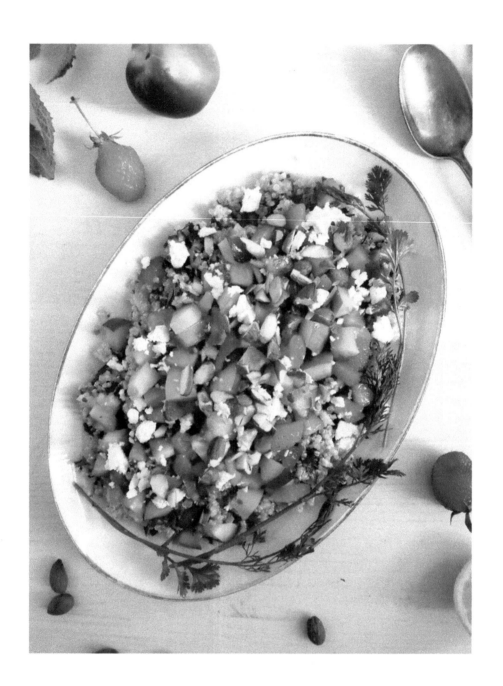

TABLE OF CONTENTS

Moroccan salad with blood oranges, olives, almond and mint

Ingredients

- 1 teaspoon of honey , maple
- 1 ¾ cups of water
- Pinch of salt
- 12 fresh mint leaves, torn
- 2 green onions, sliced diagonally
- 1 tablespoon of red wine vinegar
- 1 cup of rinsed quinoa
- ¼ cup of thinly sliced Kalamata olives
- cracked pepper and salt to taste
- ¼ cup of toasted slivered
- 3 blood oranges- divided
- ¼ cup of olive oil

Directions

1. Boil quinoa in salted water in a medium pot on the stove.
2. Lower heat once boiling, cover and cook for15 minutes.
3. In a medium bowl, add sliced green onions with sliced olives, and 2 oranges.

4. Toss the quinoa in the bowl with the oranges.
5. Dress with 4 tablespoons of olive oil , zest and juice of the remaining orange, and honey . Stir.
6. Taste and adjust accordingly.
7. Scatter with toasted slivered almonds and fresh torn mint leaves.
8. Serve and enjoy warm or chilled.

Warm grape and radicchio salad

The warm grape and radicchio salad recipe is carefully charred under the grill with incredible fresh balsamic and honey for a sweeter taste.

Ingredients

- 30g of rocket
- 200g of seedless red grapes
- 1 radicchio or 2 red chicory
- 1 tablespoon of runny honey
- 2 tablespoons of balsamic vinegar
- Olive oil
- 2 cloves of garlic
- 2 sprigs of fresh rosemary
- 2 heaped tablespoons of pine nuts

Directions

1. Place grapes on a griddle pan over a high heat let grill for 5 minutes.
2. Transfer in a large salad bowl.
3. Working in batches, grill, char the radicchio to soften on both sides.

4. Add to the bowl.
5. Add garlic, rosemary leaves, pine nuts, and oil in the still-hot griddle pan.
6. Add the balsamic vinegar together with the honey. Toss.
7. Seasoning with sea salt and black pepper.
8. Let settle for 10 minutes, then toss.
9. Serve and enjoy.

Nordic nicoise salad

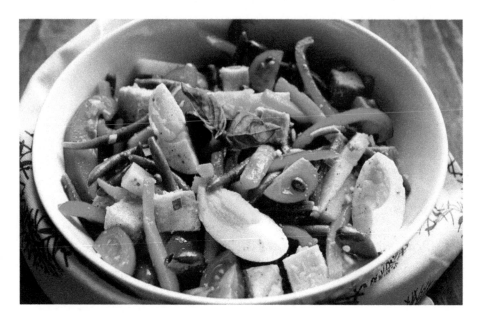

Ingredients

- 2 teaspoons of fresh grated
- 1 tablespoon of chopped fresh dill
- 2 eggs
- 1 cup of snap peas
- 1 cucumber
- Pinch sugar
- 1 tablespoon of finely chopped shallot
- 4 radishes
- 6 ounces of smoked trout
- 1 tablespoon of capers
- 2 tablespoons of fresh dill

- ¼ cup of olive oil
- 2 tablespoons of champagne vinegar
- 8 baby potatoes
- 1 teaspoon of wholegrain mustard
- 1 bunch watercress
- ¼ teaspoon of salt
- ¼ teaspoon of white pepper

Directions

1. Boil potatoes, let simmer until tender in 20 minutes.
2. Add the snap peas in the same water during the last minute.
3. Drain. Rinse under cold water.
4. Boil the eggs.
5. Stir in olive oil, champagne vinegar, mustard, shallot, dill, salt, sugar, white pepper, and horseradish, tasting and adjust.
6. Serve and enjoy with the vegetables salad.

Roasted black bean burgers

The roasted black bean burger features variety of fruits and vegetables typically mango, avocado, tabasco, tomatoes among others, making a perfect Mediterranean Sea diet.

Ingredients

- 1 ripe avocado
- 1½ red onions
- 200g of mixed mushrooms
- Chipotle tabasco sauce
- 4 tablespoons of natural yoghurt
- 100g of rye bread
- Ground coriander
- 1 x 400 g tin of black beans
- 4 sprigs of fresh coriander
- Olive oil
- 40g of mature cheddar cheese
- 1 ripe mango
- 4 soft rolls
- 100g of ripe cherry tomatoes
- 1 lime

Directions

1. Preheat the oven ready to 400°F.
2. Place 1 onion in a food processor with rye bread mushrooms, and ground coriander process until fine.
3. Drain, pulse in the black beans
4. Season lightly with sea salt and black pepper.
5. Divide into 4 and shape into patties.
6. Rub with oil and dust with ground coriander.
7. Transfer to oiled baking tray let roast for 25 minutes, until dark and crispy.
8. Top with the Cheddar, then warm the rolls.
9. Combine the onions and tomatoes in a bowl.
10. Squeeze over the lime juice with a bit of Tabasco.
11. Season to taste.
12. Halve the warm rolls and divide the yoghurt between the bases, and half of the salsa, avocado, mango, and coriander leaves.
13. Top with the burgers and the balance of salsa and press down lightly.
14. Serve and enjoy.

Brilliant bhaji burger

Ingredients

- 2 fresh green chilies
- 75g of paneer cheese
- 200g of butternut squash
- Mango chutney
- 4cm piece of ginger
- 100g of plain flour
- 1 lime
- 2 teaspoons of Rogan josh curry paste
- 2 cloves of garlic
- 2 uncooked poppadum
- Olive oil
- 4 soft burger buns
- 1 red onion
- 1 big bunch of fresh coriander
- 75g of natural yoghurt
- 1 baby gem lettuce

Directions

1. Combine onion, garlic, chilies, and coriander stalks in a bowl.
2. Add paneer with squash, ginger.

3. Sprinkle in the flour and a pinch of sea salt and black pepper.

4. Squeeze over the lime juice.

5. Add the curry paste and water, mix.

6. Drizzle 2 tablespoons of oil into a large non-stick frying pan over a medium heat.

7. Divide the mixture into 4 portions and place in the pan.

8. Let fry for 16 minutes, turning every few minutes.

9. Then pound most of the coriander leaves to a paste in a pestle, muddle in the yoghurt, season.

10. Divide the coriander yoghurt between the bases and inside bun-lids, then break up the poppadoms and sprinkle over.

11. Place a crispy bhaji burger on top of each bun-base.

12. Add a dollop of mango chutney, coriander leaves, and the lettuce.

13. Serve and enjoy chilled.

Summer Tagliatelle

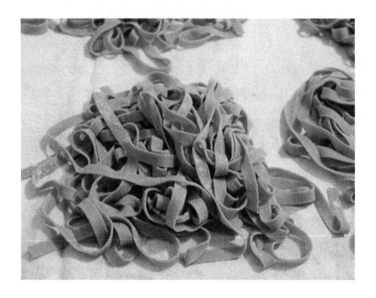

Ingredients

- 1 potato
- ½ a clove of garlic
- 200g of delicate summer vegetables
- 50g of blanched almonds
- 300g of Tagliatelle
- Extra virgin olive oil
- 25g of Parmesan cheese
- ¼ of a lemon
- 1 bunch of fresh basil
- 125g of green beans

Directions

1. Place most of the basil leaves into a pestle pulse to a paste with a pinch of sea salt.
2. Add in the garlic with pounded almonds until fine.
3. Muddle in 4 tablespoons of oil with parmesan, squeeze of lemon juice.
4. Season accordingly.
5. Place sliced potatoes and beans in a pan of boiling salted water with Tagliatelle.
6. Let cook as per the pasta packet Directions.
7. Add delicate summer vegetables to the pan for the last 3 minutes.
8. Drain, and keep some cooking water, then toss with the pesto, loosening with a splash of reserved water.
9. Drizzle with 1 tablespoon of oil, complete with basil.
10. Serve and enjoy with crunchy salad.

Roasted tomato risotto

Ingredients

- 450g of Arborio risotto rice
- 80g of Parmesan cheese
- 1 bulb of fennel
- 1 bulb of garlic
- ½ a bunch of fresh thyme
- 150ml of dry white vermouth
- Olive oil
- 1.2 liters of organic vegetable stock
- 1 onion
- 2 knobs of unsalted butter
- 6 large ripe tomatoes

Directions

1. Preheat the oven ready to 350°F.
2. Remove tomatoes seeds, place in a snug-fitting baking dish with cut sides up with garlic bulb.
3. Spread with thyme sprigs.
4. Drizzle with 1 tablespoon of oil.
5. Season with sea salt, let roast until starting to burst open.
6. Bring the stock to a simmer.

7. Place onions with olive oil and knob of butter in a large pan on a medium heat. butter.

8. Cook until softened, stirring occasionally.

9. Stir in the rice, toast for 2 minutes.

10. Pour in the vermouth, stir until absorbed.

11. Add the stock let it be fully absorbed, then add another, stirring constantly until the rice is cooked in 18 minutes.

12. Beat in the remaining knob of butter, Parmesan.

13. Season and turn off the heat.

14. Let rest for 2 minutes.

15. Divide the risotto between warm plates, place a tomato in the center with sweet garlic and the herby fennel.

16. Serve and enjoy.

Veggie pad Thai

Ingredients

- 320g of crunchy vegetables
- Sesame oil
- Olive oil
- 80g of silken tofu
- Low-salt soy sauce
- 150g of rice noodles
- ½ a mixed bunch of fresh basil, mint and coriander
- 2 teaspoons of tamarind paste
- 2 cloves of garlic
- ½ a cos lettuce
- 2 teaspoons of sweet chili sauce
- 2 limes
- 20g of unsalted peanuts
- 1 shallot
- 80g of beansprouts
- 2 large free-range eggs
- Dried chili flakes

Directions

1. Start by cook the noodles according to the packet Directions.
2. Drain any excess water, toss with 1 teaspoon of sesame oil.
3. Toast the peanuts in a large non-stick frying pan on a medium heat until golden.
4. Blend in a pestle until fine, place into a bowl.
5. Bash the garlic to a paste with the tofu.
6. Add sesame oil with soy, tamarind paste, and chili sauce.
7. Muddle in half the lime juice.
8. Place slices of shallot in a frying pan over a high heat.
9. Dry-fry the crunchy veggies for 4 minutes.
10. Add the noodles together with sauce, beansprouts, and splash of water, toss over heat for 1 minute.
11. Wipe out the pan, crack in the eggs let cook in a little olive oil, sprinkled with a pinch of chili flakes.
12. Place lettuce in the bowls with eggs on top and pick over the herbs.
13. Serve and enjoy with lime wedges.

Pea and ricotta stuffed courgettes

Ingredients

- 2 cloves of garlic
- 4 sprigs of fresh mint
- olive oil
- 100g of ricotta cheese
- 50g of mature Cheddar cheese
- 300g of basmati rice
- 1 lemon
- 8 baby courgettes, with flowers
- 400g of ripe cherry tomatoes
- red wine vinegar
- 150g of fresh or frozen peas
- 4 spring onions
- 8 black olives
- 1 fresh red chili

Directions

1. Preheat the oven ready to 400°F.
2. Process the mint leaves in a food processor with peas, ricotta, and Cheddar.

3. Squeeze in the lemon juice with black pepper, blend until smooth.

4. Taste and adjust the seasoning.

5. Fill each courgette flower with the mixture, seal the petals.

6. Place the tomatoes, onions, and olives roasting tray.

7. Drizzle with 2 tablespoons each of oil and vinegar, season with pepper.

8. Stir in the rice and boiling water, bring to the boil, stirring occasionally.

9. Bake the courgettes inside rice for 20 minutes until golden.

10. Serve and enjoy with summery salad

Veggie pasties

Ingredients

- 1 large free-range egg
- 250g of unsalted butter
- 200g of swede
- 1 pinch of dried rosemary
- 400g of potatoes
- 500g of strong flour
- 1 onion
- 500g of mixed mushrooms

Directions

1. Tear the mushrooms into a bowl, scatter over 15g of sea salt, leave for 30 minutes, scrunching occasionally.
2. Place flour with a pinch of salt into a bowl.
3. Rub in the butter.
4. Make a well in the middle, pour in cold water, mix, pat dry.
5. Wrap in Clingfilm and refrigerate for 1 hour.
6. Squeeze to salty liquid after 30 minutes.
7. Mix the veggies with the mushrooms, rosemary and pinches of black pepper.
8. Preheat the oven to 350°F.

9. Divide the pastry into 8, then roll out into rounds.
10. Divide up the filling, then scrunch and pile it to one side of the middle.
11. Brush the exposed pastry with beaten egg, fold over and press the edges down, seal with your thumb. Egg wash.
12. Place on a lined baking sheet let bake for 40 minutes.
13. Serve and enjoy with watercress.

Asparagus quiche and soup

Ingredients

- 1.5 liters of organic vegetable stock
- 125g of whole meal flour
- 2 onions
- 150g of mature Cheddar cheese
- 125g of unsalted butter
- 7 large free-range eggs
- 1kg of asparagus
- 150g of ricotta cheese
- Olive oil
- 125g of plain flour
- 2 large potatoes
- ½ a bunch of fresh thyme

Directions

1. Preheat the oven to 350°F.
2. Put flours into a bowl with pinch of sea salt, rub in the butter.
3. Make a well in the middle, crack in one of the eggs, mix with cold water, pat dry and bring together.
4. Place between two large sheets of greaseproof paper, flatten, chill for 30 minutes.

5. Roll out the pastry between the sheets, line a loose-bottomed tart tin with the pastry, bake for 20 minutes.

6. Place asparagus and oil in a large pan over a medium heat.

7. Add the potatoes with onions, thyme leaves cook until lightly golden, stirring regularly.

8. Pour in the stock, boil, then simmer for 15 minutes.

9. Blend until smooth, sieve.

10. Season to taste with salt and black pepper.

11. Beat the remaining eggs in a bowl with a pinch of salt and pepper.

12. Add the ricotta with Cheddar and remaining thyme leaves.

13. Stir the asparagus into the egg mixture and tip into the tart case.

14. Let bake for 40 minutes.

15. Serve and enjoy.

Summer vegetable blanket pie

Ingredients

- 320g of ripe cherry tomatoes
- 4 cloves of garlic
- 1 tablespoon of fennel seeds
- Olive oil
- 1 pinch of saffron
- 320g of potatoes
- 320g of butternut squash
- 320g of courgettes
- 1 tablespoon of sesame seeds
- ½ x 700g jar of chickpeas
- 1 large leek
- Extra virgin olive oil
- 8 sheets of filo pastry
- 1 preserved lemon
- 1 tablespoon of red wine vinegar
- 400g of natural yoghurt
- 1 teaspoon of rose harissa
- 50g of dried sour cherries

Directions

1. Sieve the yogurt through into a bowl, then leave to drain.

2. Season the tomatoes with sea salt and black pepper.

3. Drizzle with extra virgin olive oil and the vinegar, then toss, let macerate.

4. Preheat the oven to 375°F.

5. Place garlic slices in a large frying pan on a medium heat with the fennel seeds and olive oil.

6. Fry briefly, stirring regularly.

7. Add potatoes, leek, and courgette let cook covered for 15 minutes.

8. Add the chickpeas, season with a pinch of salt and pepper.

9. Add lemon to the pan with a drizzle of juice from the jar, and the harissa.

10. Continue to fry for 15 more minutes, stirring occasionally.

11. Cover the sour cherries and saffron with boiling water, add tomatoes, reserving the macerating juices.

12. Lay the filo out flat, then brush with tomato juices.

13. Scatter over the sesame seeds and bake for 25 minutes

14. Serve and enjoy with the pie.

Allotment cottage pie

The delicious taste of the allotment cottage pie will surprise anyone's taste buds.

It is fully packed with variety of nutrients and a perfect Mediterranean Sea diet choice.

Ingredients

- 1 teaspoon of Marmite
- 2 large leeks
- 3 carrots
- 1 x 400g tin of green lentils
- 1 splash of semi-skimmed milk
- 10g of dried porcini mushrooms
- 500g of swede
- 500g of celeriac
- Olive oil
- 3 sprigs of fresh rosemary
- 1 onion
- 3 tablespoons of tomato purée
- 1 teaspoon cumin seeds
- 2kg of potatoes
- 40g of unsalted butter

Directions

1. In a blender, cover the porcini with hot water.
2. Drizzle oil into a large casserole pan over a medium heat.
3. Fry the rosemary for 1 minute to crisp up.
4. Add the cumin seeds together with prepared veggies to flavored oil.
5. Season with sea salt and black pepper, cook for 30 minutes, stirring regularly.
6. Cook the potatoes in a pan of boiling salted water until tender.
7. Drain and mash with butter and milk, then season.
8. Preheat the oven to 375°F.
9. Add onions, marmite, tomato puree, blend until smooth.
10. Pour into the veggie pan and cook for 20 minutes, stirring regularly.
11. Place the lentils into the veg pan, boil, season to taste.
12. Spoon over the mash, place on a tray.
13. Let bake for 30 minutes, or until bubbling at the edges.
14. Sprinkle over the crispy rosemary.
15. Serve and enjoy with seasonal greens.

Sticky onion tart

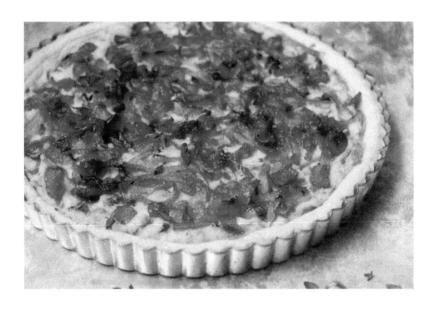

The stick onion tart is quite flavorful with garlic and the onion itself. Above and beyond, this recipe is easy to make.

Ingredients

- 4 tablespoons of cider vinegar
- 4 medium onions
- 320g of sheet of all-butter puff pastry
- 50g of unsalted butter

- 8 cloves of garlic
- 4 sprigs of fresh thyme
- 4 fresh bay leaves
- 2 tablespoons of soft dark brown sugar

Directions

1. Preheat the oven ready to 425°F.
2. Place butter in an ovenproof frying pan on a medium heat.
3. Add thyme leaves with the bay, sugar, vinegar, and water.
4. Place the onion halves in the pan, cut side down with garlic in between.
5. Season with sea salt and black pepper.
6. Cover, over low heat and steam for 10 minutes to soften the onions, uncover cook until liquid starts to caramelize.
7. Place the pastry over the onions, placed to the edge of the pan.
8. Let bake for 35 minutes, until golden brown.
9. Serve and enjoy.

Tomato curry

Ingredients

- 2 teaspoons of mango chutney
- 1 onion
- 1.2kg of ripe mixed tomatoes
- 1 pinch of saffron
- 1 teaspoon of mustard seeds
- 1 teaspoon of fenugreek seeds
- 1 x 400g tin of light coconut milk
- 20g of flaked almonds
- 4 cloves of garlic
- 1 teaspoon of cumin seeds
- 4cm piece of ginger
- 2 fresh red chilies
- Olive oil
- 1 handful of fresh curry leaves

Directions

1. Prick the tomatoes, plunge into fast-boiling water briefly.
2. Peel the skin.
3. Cover the saffron with boiling water and leave to infuse.
4. Toast the almonds in a large non-stick frying pan over a medium heat until golden.

5. Transfer to a small bowl and place the pan back on the heat.

6. Drizzle 1 tablespoon of oil into the pan, add curry leaves with all the spices.

7. Add onions with garlic, ginger, and chili to the pan, let fry for 3 minutes, stirring constantly.

8. Add the tomatoes with the coconut milk and saffron water, let simmer for 20 minutes covered.

9. Add mango chutney halfway.

10. Season to taste with sea salt and black pepper, scatter over the almonds.

11. Serve and enjoy with fluffy rice.

Vegetable chili

Ingredients

- 2 sweet potatoes
- 1 x 400g tin of cannellini beans
- 3 mixed-color peppers
- 4 large ripe tomatoes
- 1 lemon
- 1 bunch of fresh mint
- 4 tablespoons of natural yoghurt
- Olive oil
- 1 teaspoon of cumin seeds
- 1 teaspoon of smoked paprika
- 2 red onions
- 4 small flour tortillas
- 4 cloves of garlic
- Hot chili sauce
- 250g of black rice

Directions

1. Preheat a griddle pan ready to high temperature.
2. Drizzle 1 tablespoon of oil into a large casserole pan over a medium-low heat.

3. Stir in the cumin with paprika, garlic, lemon zest, and grilled vegetables, stirring regularly.

4. Add the beans and water, add chili sauce.

5. Season with sea salt and black pepper let simmer for 30 minutes.

6. Cook the rice in a pan of boiling salted water according to the packet Directions.

7. Pick 2 sprigs of mint leaves and chop with the salsa veggie, toss with the lemon juice.

8. Season to taste with salt and pepper.

9. Warm the tortillas on the griddle and ripple shakes of chili sauce through the yoghurt.

10. Serve and enjoy with black rice.

Chicken and vegetable stir-fry

Ingredients

- 2 carrots
- ½ of a red onion
- 1 red pepper
- 80g of purple sprouting broccoli
- 1 tablespoon of reduced-salt soy sauce
- 80g of mixed mushrooms
- 1 free-range chicken breast
- 1 teaspoon of sesame seeds
- 1 tablespoon of sesame oil
- 4cm of piece of ginger
- 1 teaspoon of Chinese five-spice
- 1 teaspoon of vegetable oil
- Sprigs of fresh coriander
- 1 fresh red chili
- 1 clove of garlic
- 130g of baby corn
- 80g of mange tout
- 2 whole wheat noodle nests
- 1 tablespoon of black bean sauce

Directions

1. Place the chicken into a bowl with the Chinese five-spice and sesame oil, toss.
2. Place a large non-stick frying pan over a medium-high heat with the vegetable oil.
3. Add the garlic together with the ginger and chili, toss briefly.
4. Add the chicken let stir-fry for 2 minutes until golden.
5. Add all the vegetables, let stir-fry for more 4 minutes.
6. Cook the noodles as instructed on the package in a large pan of boiling salted water.
7. Transfer the noodles to the pan, add soy with black bean sauce, toss to coat.
8. Scatter over the sesame seeds and coriander.
9. Serve and enjoy.

Roasted vegetable roots

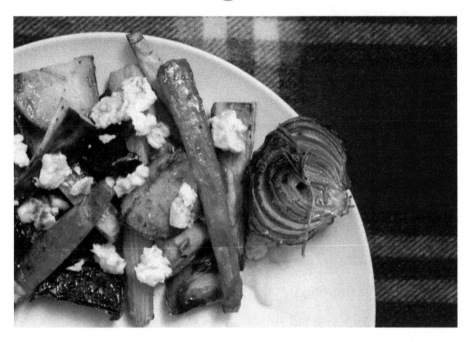

Much as there are various ways one can roast veggies, the Mediterranean style is mega for a delicious and aromatic flavor with garlic taking the lead.

Ingredients

- 12 parsnips
- 3kg of potatoes
- 16 carrots
- ½ a bunch of fresh rosemary
- 1 bulb of garlic

Directions

1. Begin by preheat your oven ready to 375°F.
2. Cook potatoes with parsnips and carrots in a large pan of boiling salted water for 8 minutes.
3. Drain any excess water in a colander let steam dry.
4. Remove the carrots and parsnips put to one side, shakes the colander.
5. Add 4 tablespoons of olive oil to two large roasting trays.
6. Season each with sea salt and black pepper.
7. Squash the garlic bulb, divide between the trays with the rosemary sprigs.
8. Place in the veggies, red wine vinegar, toss to coat.
9. Let roast for 40 minutes.
10. Remove and squash with a fish slice to burst the skins.
11. Place back in the oven for 20 minutes.
12. Serve and enjoy.

Pina colada fro-yo

Ingredients

- 6 ice cream scones
- 500g of frozen chopped tropical fruits
- 250g of Greek-style coconut yoghurt
- 75g of dried tropical fruit

Directions

1. Start by adding the yoghurt and frozen fruit to a food processor.
2. Blend until smooth
3. Chop and fold through most of the dried fruit, saving some for serving.
4. Spoon the mixture into a piping bag with a large star-shaped nozzle.
5. Freeze for about 30 minutes.
6. Pipe the fruity fro-yo into your ice cream cones and scatter over the reserved dried fruit.
7. Serve and enjoy.

Plum sorbet

Ingredients

- 10 plums
- ½ of a lemon
- 200g of sugar
- 1 free-range egg white

Directions

1. Combine the plums together with 100g of sugar in a large bowl.
2. Cover tightly with Clingfilm, set over a pan of simmering water to release the plum juices for about 30 minutes.
3. Sieve the plums to release the juice.
4. Make a sugar syrup by dissolving the remaining sugar in 100ml of boiling water.
5. Pour 100ml into the plum juice.
6. Beat the egg white until frothy.
7. add in the lemon juice, stir into the plum juice.
8. Taste, and adjust accordingly.
9. Serve and enjoy.

Plum lattice pie

Ingredients

- 3 tablespoons of corn flour
- 1 teaspoon of cinnamon
- 275g of plain flour
- 50g of butter
- 2 tablespoons of icing sugar
- ½ teaspoon of ground ginger
- 130g of butter
- 3 medium free-range egg yolks
- 100g of caster sugar
- Milk
- caster sugar
- 50g of flaked almonds
- 10 plums

Directions

1. Preheat the oven to 400°F.
2. Combine the flour together with the icing sugar, and a pinch of sea salt into a food processor.
3. Add the butter, let blend until fine like breadcrumbs.
4. Add 2 egg yolks with ice-cold water, pulse until you have a dough.

5. Divide into two pieces, roll out into discs wrapping both in Clingfilm and chill in the fridge for 30 minutes.

6. Roll out the larger piece of pastry and press into a pie tin let chill in the fridge.

7. Roll out the remaining disc and cut out eight long, even strips, each 2.5cm wide.

8. Toast the almonds in a dry frying pan until golden.

9. Place all ingredients in a large bowl and stir well.

10. Pile the fruit mixture into the pie base.

11. Then, beat the remaining egg yolk with a splash of milk.

12. Brush the edges of the pastry with it.

13. Arrange, weave the pastry strips in a lattice pattern on top of the pie.

14. Brush the pie with the egg wash and sprinkle with sugar.

15. Chill in the fridge for 30 minutes.

16. Let bake for 20 minutes, checking occasionally.

17. Lower the heat to medium, let bake for 30 minutes more covered with a foil.

18. Remove, sprinkle with extra sugar and let set for 3 hours.

19. Serve and enjoy.

Soaked pistachio and citrus cake

Ingredients

- 1 teaspoon of dried mint
- 25g of pistachios
- 75g of unsalted butter
- 4 large free-range eggs
- 50g of no-peel orange marmalade
- 250g of sugar
- 1 lemon
- 2 lemons
- 100g of ground pistachios
- 100g of fine semolina

1. **Directions**
2. Preheat your oven ready to 350°F.
3. Grease and line a cake tin.
4. Then, Melt butter over a low heat, set aside.
5. In an electric mixer, beat the egg yolks with the sugar until creamy.
6. Add the pistachios and semolina as the mixer runs, melted butter, lemon zest, marmalade, and sea salt. Blend smooth.
7. In a separate bowl, whisk the egg whites.

8. Fold into pistachio mixture in three additions.

9. Pour the batter into the prepared tin.

10. Let bake for 30 minutes.

11. Combine the lemon juice with sugar in a saucepan over a medium heat until the sugar has dissolved.

12. Remove, set aside.

13. Pour the syrup over the cake while warm.

14. Sprinkle with the dried mint, chop, scatter over the pistachios.

15. Serve slices with a spoonful of Greek yoghurt when cooled completely.

Asian style watermelon salad

This Asian style watermelon salad is a refreshing recipe mainly for the summer season, but also for any other season.

It features radishes, fresh mint flavors with garlic, dressing with chili hum.

Ingredients

- 2 limes
- 20g of sesame seeds
- ½ of a watermelon
- 1 tablespoon low-salt soy sauce
- 5cm piece of ginger
- 1 bunch of breakfast radishes
- 2 fresh red chilies
- ½ a bunch of fresh mint
- 1 tablespoon of sesame oil
- 1 lime
- ½ a clove of garlic

Directions

1. Over a medium heat, toast the sesame seeds in a hot dry pan briefly. Set aside.
2. Prepare the ginger, garlic, and chili in a jar.
3. Squeeze in the lime juice.
4. Then add the soy and oil, cover, shake to combine.
5. Combine the watermelon together with the radishes in a bowl.
6. Add over the dressing, scatter over the sliced mint, toss to combine.
7. Scattering with a toasted sesame seeds and the baby mint leaves.
8. Serve and enjoy, then serve with lime wedges.

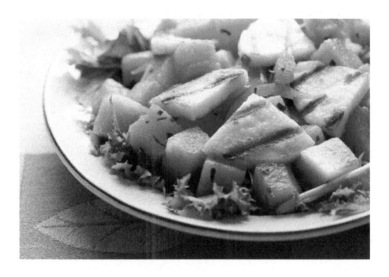

Rainbow jelly

This is a veggie packed recipe with a variety of fruits with various flavors and fresh fruity juice.

This will surprise your taste buds.

Ingredients

- vegetable oil
- 4 packets of jelly

Directions

1. Begin by wiping inside of the jelly mold with a tiny bit of oil.
2. Make jelly layer as per the packet Directions, pour into your mold.
3. Refrigerate for 20 minutes.
4. Crack on with the next colored jelly, pour it into your mold when the previous layer is just firm enough.
5. Repeat process for all the layers and color of jelly while your mold is in the fridge.
6. Serve and enjoy.

Blackberry fool

Ingredients

- 330ml of double cream
- 1 vanilla pod
- 500g of blackberries
- 1 lemon
- 200ml of fat-free Greek yoghurt
- 100g of caster sugar

Directions

1. Prepare and place the vanilla in a large pan together with the berries, sugar, and lemon juice.
2. Boil over a medium heat.
3. Let simmer for 4 minutes or until the syrupy and the berries are soft. Set aside to cool.
4. In a large bowl, whisk the cream to form peaks.
5. Fold through the yogurt and swirl through the syrup.
6. Layer the rest of the syrup and cream in dessert glasses
7. Serve and enjoy garnished with a syrup and fresh berries.

Baked berries with brandy mascarpone

Ingredients

- 250g of mascarpone
- 100ml of brandy
- 4 tablespoons of soft dark brown sugar
- 750g of mixed berries

Directions

1. Preheat your grill ready to full whack.
2. In a bowl, mix the berries together with the brandy and sugar.
3. Pour into a dish, dot with the mascarpone.
4. Then, sprinkle over the rest of the sugar.
5. Place under grill for 5 minutes.
6. Serve and enjoy.

Hot cross muffins

Ingredients

- 175g of mixed dried fruit
- ¼ teaspoon of sea salt
- 225g of unsalted butter preferably at room temperature
- 3 large free-range eggs
- 50g of dried cranberries
- 100g of icing sugar
- 150g of ground almonds
- 100g of buckwheat flour
- 1 teaspoon of ground mixed spice
- 1 eating apple
- 200g of light of Muscovado sugar
- 1½ teaspoons of gluten-free baking powder
- 1 large orange

Directions

1. Heat your oven ready to 380°F.
2. Line two muffin trays with paper cases.
3. In a large bowl, beat the butter together with sugar in an electric beater until fluffy.
4. Then, combine the almonds together with the flour, mixed spice, baking powder, and salt in a bowl.

5. Add on top of the creamed butter and sugar.

6. Add the orange zest together with juice and the eggs to the bowl.

7. Mix together until you have a thick batter.

8. Stir in the dried fruit, cranberries, and apple.

9. Dollop the mixture into the muffin cases.

10. Let bake for 35 minutes, lower the heat to medium.

11. Continue to bake for 25 minutes, until the muffins are golden.

12. Let cool in the tin for 15 minutes, shift to a cooling rack.

13. Mix the icing sugar with 5 teaspoons of the orange juice.

14. Spoon into a piping bag with a round nozzle.

15. Pipe crosses onto each muffin, then dust with extra icing sugar.

16. Let settle, serve and enjoy.

Poached peaches or apricots and lemon grass

This recipe has the freshest flavor elevated with the lemon grass.

It will definitely keep you wanting more for a perfect Mediterranean Sea diet.

Ingredients

- 50g of sugar
- 2 stalks of lemongrass
- 8 peaches or 12 apricots

Directions

1. Prepare the lemongrass and place in a small pan.
2. Heat sugar and water in the pan with the lemongrass over a medium heat to dissolve the sugar.
3. Add the peaches or apricots, press a circle of greaseproof paper down on top to cover the fruit.
4. Simmer gently for 5 minutes for apricot and 12 minutes for peaches.
5. Cool in a bowl.
6. Serve and enjoy.

Vegan toffee apple upside down cake

The topping used in this recipe mainly the apples make this meal delicious and a perfect choice for a Mediterranean Sea diet with its health benefits.

Ingredients

- 85g of shelled walnuts
- 195g of muscovado sugar
- 180g of plain flour
- 1 teaspoon of bicarbonate of soda
- 25g of vegan margarine
- 1 lemon
- 1½ teaspoons of mixed spice
- 80ml of sunflower oil
- 1 teaspoon of vinegar
- 3 dessert apples

Directions

1. Grate 2 apples and slice the others.
2. Melt sugar together with the margarine in a pan.

3. Pour into the prepared tin.
4. Top with the sliced apple in a single layer.
5. Then, combine the flour together with the sugar, bicarbonate of soda, and mixed spice in a bowl.
6. In another separate bowl, combine the oil together with water, vinegar, grated apple, and lemon zest.
7. Thoroughly mix the dry ingredients with the wet.
8. Stir in chopped walnuts.
9. Pour over the layer of apples in the cake tin.
10. Let bake for 30 minutes, let cool for 5 minutes.
11. Serve and enjoy.

Pomegranate and clementine sorbet

Ingredient

- 5 clementine
- 1 lemon
- 500ml of fresh pomegranate juice
- 50g of granulated sugar

Directions

1. Add sugar and water in a pan over a low heat.
2. Stir until the sugar has dissolved, place into a jug.
3. Squeeze in the clementine and lemon juice into the jug
4. Add the pomegranate juice and chill in the fridge, then freeze.
5. When already in ice crystals, whisk, return to the freezer.
6. Repeat 4 times until you have a smooth sorbet.
7. Blend in a food processor, freeze again until ready to serve.
8. Enjoy.

Passion-berry choux buns

The balance and aromatic flavors of the passion fruit and berries elevates the taste of this recipe beyond your imagination for a Mediterranean Sea diet.

Ingredients

- 300g of raspberries
- Caster sugar
- 1 lemon
- 25g of butter
- 4 medium free-range eggs
- 1 large free-range egg
- 3 large free-range egg yolks
- 125ml of Greek yoghurt
- ½ teaspoon of vanilla bean paste
- 125ml of double cream
- 50g of butter
- 4 large passion fruit
- 75ml of whole milk
- 250g of fondant icing sugar
- 100g of plain flour

Directions

1. Place the berries into a saucepan together with 1 tablespoon of the sugar, lemon juice, and splash of water.
2. Let cook for 5 minutes over a low heat sieving into a heatproof bowl.
3. Mix the remaining sugar into the raspberries.
4. Add the butter, over simmering water until melted.
5. In another separate bowl, beat the egg and vanilla bean paste.
6. Whisk in 3 tablespoons of the warm raspberry mixture to loosen, mix into the raspberry in the bowl.
7. Cook over the simmering water for 10 minutes, stirring often.
8. Strain the mixture into a clean bowl, cover with Clingfilm, let cool.
9. Preheat your oven to 360°F.
10. Dice, add butter to a pan together with milk and water.
11. Place over low heat to melt the butter, raise heat to bring the mixture to a rolling boil.
12. Remove pan from the hob.
13. Place and beat in the flour with sugar and a pinch of sea salt until smooth.
14. Dry out the mixture a little.
15. Beat the eggs, add to the choux mixture, mix well.
16. Line a baking tray with greaseproof paper, add choux batter onto it.

17. Let bake for 20 minutes.

18. Release the steam by piercing at the bottom of each burn.

19. Cool on a wire rack.

20. In another bowl, whip the double cream with the Greek yoghurt until it holds firm peaks.

21. Fold in the raspberry curd until it holds soft peaks.

22. Scoop the filling into a piping bag with a plain nozzle.

23. Cut a small hole underneath each choux bun and fill with the raspberry cream.

24. Scoop passion fruit pulp into a sieve set over a bowl.

25. Whisk the fondant icing sugar into the juice until smooth.

26. Place passion fruit icing over each bun, let set for 5 minutes.

27. Serve and enjoy.

Four-grain coconut porridge with autumnal fruit

A combination of variety of grains makes this Mediterranean Sea diet recipe an energy powerhouse flavored with the coconut, you do not have to worry about your breakfast and lunch or dinner.

Ingredients

- 100g of oat bran
- 350ml of unsweetened coconut milk
- 1 orange
- Runny honey
- 10 g of oatmeal
- 1 vanilla pod
- 2 pears
- 100g of quinoa
- 1 handful of blackberries
- 1 tablespoon of hazelnuts
- 200g of porridge mix
- 1 tablespoon of chia seeds
- 200g of large porridge oats

Directions

1. Combine porridge oats, oat bran, oat meal, and quinoa in an airtight container.
2. Place the porridge mix in a medium saucepan.
3. Add the coconut milk, hot water, and the orange zest.
4. Add vanilla pod and seeds to the pan.
5. Over a medium heat, let cook for 20 minutes, stirring continuously.
6. Grate the pears into a bowl, add sliced blackberries. Toss.
7. Toast the hazelnuts in a dry frying pan over a medium heat, chop.
8. Remove vanilla pod from the pan.
9. Serve and enjoy with fruit, chia seeds, and hazelnuts.

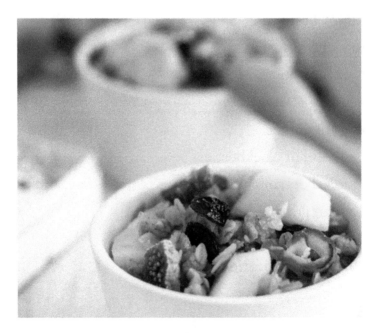

Stuffed fruit crumble

Ingredients

- 1 large free-range egg white
- 1 orange
- ½ of a vanilla pod
- 75g of caster sugar
- 4 large plums
- 70g of desiccated coconut
- 3 cardamom pods

Directions

1. Preheat your oven ready to 380°F.
2. Place cardamom powder into a bowl.
3. Add the vanilla flesh to bowl.
4. Mix in the sugar together with the egg white, coconut, all the orange zest and half the juice.
5. Place the plums cut-side up on a baking tray.
6. Pile the coconut mixture into the holes
7. Let bake for 18 minutes.
8. Serve and enjoy with vanilla ice cream.

Pear and ginger pudding

Ingredients

- 1 ripe pear
- Golden syrup
- 1 large free-range egg
- 55g of self-rising flour
- 1 piece of stem ginger in syrup
- 55g of unsalted butter
- 55g of caster sugar
- 1 orange

Directions

1. Place 2 teacups upside down on greaseproof paper, draw round them.
2. Cut out the circles.
3. Grease one side with butter, then grease the inside of the teacups.
4. Using a food processor, process the flour together with the sugar, butter, and egg.
5. Add the ginger, orange zest, pulse twice.
6. Pour a small golden syrup into the base of each cup, top with half the chopped pear each.

7. Divide the batter between the two cups, then lightly press a circle of paper on top, butter-side down.

8. Let cook in the microwave, full power for 4 minutes.

9. Let cool.

10. Serve and enjoy with lashings of hot custard.

Berry good pancakes

Ingredients

- 1 handful of blueberries
- 1 cup self-rising flour
- 6 slices of streaky bacon
- 1 teaspoon baking powder
- 1 large free-range egg
- 20g of butter
- 1 cup of milk

Directions

1. Crack the eggs, fill the same cup with flour.
2. Add to the bowl. Toss in the baking powder.
3. Fill the cup with milk, add a tiny pinch of sea salt.
4. Whisk till smooth. Cover the bowl in Clingfilm and put to one side.
5. Heat a non-stick frying pan, let fry until crisp.
6. Put a large frying pan on a medium heat, melt the butter.
7. Place the pancake batter into the pan.
8. Let cook 2 minutes, until little bubbles rise up to the top. Turnover.
9. Dot a handful of blueberries across the half-cooked pancakes.

10. Transfer to a plate and cover with foil.

11. Add the remaining butter, use all the butter.

12. Serve and enjoy with the bacon.

Cranberry granola

Ingredients

- 2 tablespoons of vegetable oil
- Runny honey
- 400g of jumbo rolled oats
- 100g of seeds
- 200g of mixed nuts
- 150g of dried cranberries
- 1 teaspoon of ground cinnamon
- 500g of plain yoghurt

Directions

1. Begin by preheating your oven ready to 350°F.
2. Mix the nuts with the oats, half the cranberries, seeds, and the oil. Stir.
3. Divide between 2 baking sheets, let cook for 25 minutes till golden.
4. Mix the yoghurt together with the cinnamon.
5. Serve the granola with the yoghurt and a drizzle of honey.
6. Enjoy.

Passion fruit cairipinha

Ingredients

- 4 tablespoons of golden caster sugar
- Crushed ice
- 3 limes
- 75ml of cachaça
- 1 ripe passion fruit

Directions

1. Begin by cutting the limes into wedges.
2. Place the lime wedges except 2 with sugar in a cocktail shaker.
3. Muddle briefly to almost dissolve the sugar.
4. Add the cachaça, spoon in most of the passion fruit pulp.
5. Fill the shaker with crushed ice and shake for 1 minute.
6. Pour the cocktail into 2 glasses.
7. Use the 2 remaining lime wedges to garnish and the passion fruit pulp.
8. Serve and enjoy.

Date, cocoa and pumpkin recipe

Ingredients

- 1 teaspoon of vanilla extract
- 1 orange
- 50g of whole almonds
- 80g of Medjool dates
- 1cm piece of fresh turmeric
- ½ teaspoon of ground cinnamon
- 20g of puffed brown rice
- 1 heaped teaspoon of quality cocoa powder
- 70g of pumpkin seeds
- ½ tablespoon of Manuka honey

Directions

1. Expressly, blend 40g pumpkin seeds into a dust in a food processor.
2. Add remaining pumpkin seeds with the puffed rice in the processor, almonds, and dates. Blend to chop.
3. Add the ground turmeric, with cinnamon, cocoa powder, and a pinch of sea salt.
4. Blend again until ground
5. Add the vanilla together with the honey and half the orange juice.

6. Blend briefly.

7. Divide into 24 then roll into balls.

8. Throw into the pumpkin seed dust.

9. Shake to coat, storing them in the excess dust until needed.

10. Serve and enjoy.

Vegetable Mediterranean recipes

Vegetables are the heart and a true definition of a Mediterranean Sea diet. It is the origin of all the health benefits associated with the Mediterranean Sea diet together with the fruits that make the Mediterranean meals complete.

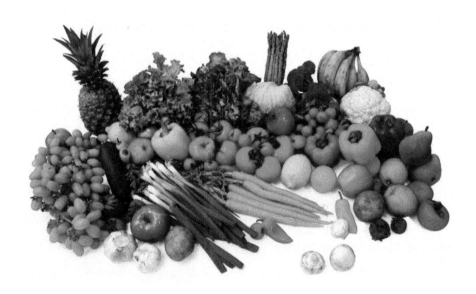

Versatile veggie chili

The versatile veggie chili recipe is quite delicious and a hearty substitution to traditional chili.

It features butternut squash, leek and spring onions for a greater flavor coupled with cayenne pepper for a perfect choice of a Mediterranean Sea diet.

Ingredients

- 1 heaped teaspoon ground cumin
- Lime or lemon juice, or vinegar
- Olive oil
- 2 mixed-color peppers
- 2 cloves of garlic
- 1 level teaspoon cayenne pepper
- 2 x 400g of tins of beans
- 1 bunch of fresh coriander
- 2 fresh mixed-color chilies
- 1 onion
- 1 level teaspoon ground cinnamon
- 2 x 400g of tins of quality plum tomatoes
- 500g of sweet potatoes

Directions

1. Preheat the oven ready to 400°F.
2. Prepare and place chopped potatoes onto a baking tray.
3. Sprinkle with a pinch of cayenne, cinnamon, cumin, sea salt and black pepper.
4. Drizzle with oil then toss to coat.
5. Let roast for 1 hour or until golden.
6. Place 2 tablespoons of oil in a large pan over a medium-high heat.
7. Add the onion together with peppers, and garlic.
8. Let cook for 5 minutes, stirring regularly.
9. Add the coriander stalks together with the chilies and spices.
10. Cook for more 10 minutes or until softened, stirring occasionally.
11. Add the beans, juice and all.
12. Tip in the tomatoes, breaking them up with the back of a spoon, stir well.
13. Let boil, lower the heat to medium-low for 30 minutes.
14. Stir the roasted sweet potato through the chili with most of the coriander leaves,
15. Taste and adjust accordingly.
16. Add a squeeze of lime or lemon juice or a swig of vinegar.
17. Serve and enjoy with yogurt or sour cream.

Classic ratatouille

Ingredients

- 2 red onions
- 4 cloves of garlic
- 2 aborigines
- 3 courgettes
- 3 red or yellow peppers
- 6 ripe tomatoes
- ½ a bunch of fresh basil
- Olive oil
- A few sprigs of fresh thyme
- 1 x 400 g tin of quality plum tomatoes
- 1 tablespoon of balsamic vinegar
- ½ of a lemon

Directions

1. Start by heating 2 tablespoons of oil in a large casserole pan over a medium heat.
2. Add the chopped aubergines together with the courgettes and peppers.
3. Let fry for 5 minutes, spoon the cooked vegetables into a large bowl.
4. Add the onion, garlic, basil stalks, and thyme leaves with another drizzle of oil to the pan.

5. Let fry for 15 minutes or until golden.

6. Return the cooked veggie to the pan.

7. Stir in the fresh and tinned tomatoes together with the balsamic and a pinch of sea salt and black pepper.

8. Cover and let simmer over a low heat for 35 minutes.

9. Tear in the basil leaves, grate in the lemon zest.

10. Taste and adjust seasoning accordingly.

11. Serve and enjoy with steamed rice.

Carrot spinach juice

Combining carrots with spinach provides a rich source of iron, calcium, and vitamins along with other mineral.

It is a tastier Mediterranean juice with a simple step-by-step method.

Ingredients

- 6 medium size carrots
- 1 large bunch of spinach
- Celery stalk
- ½ of lemon
- 1 ½ cups of water

Directions

1. Combine the carrots together with the celery stalk and all the water in a blender.
2. Blend to puree.
3. Then, add the spinach and juice of lemon, (squeeze).
4. Blend briefly, then, strain.
5. Serve and enjoy.

Fresh tomato juice

Ingredients

- Celery stalks
- Salt
- 2 ice cubes
- ¼ teaspoon of ground black pepper
- 2 carrots
- 6 ripe tomatoes

Directions

1. Place tomatoes together with the carrots and celery in a blender.
2. Blend until smooth.
3. Then, add salt with black pepper to season, mix well.
4. Add the ice cubes in serving glasses.
5. Serve and enjoy.

Aubergine parmigiana

This a great meal recipe originating from the parts of northern Italy making a perfect Mediterranean Sea diet with variety of vegetables.

It can be served perfectly with roasted fish.

Ingredients

- 1 bunch of fresh basil
- A few sprigs of fresh oregano
- 3 large firm aubergines
- 2 handfuls of dried breadcrumbs
- 150g of buffalo mozzarella
- Olive oil
- ½ a bulb of spring garlic
- 1 heaped teaspoon dried oregano
- 2 x 400g tins of quality plum tomatoes
- Wine vinegar
- 1 onion
- 3 large handfuls of parmesan cheese

Directions

1. Preheat a griddle barbecue ready.
2. Place a large pan on a medium heat with olive oil.
3. Add the onion together with the garlic and dried oregano.
4. Let cook for 10 minutes.
5. Add the tomato flesh to onion pan, stir well, cover and let simmer 15 minutes over low heat.
6. Grill the aubergines on both sides until lightly charred.
7. Season the tomato sauce with sea salt, black pepper and a tiny swig of wine vinegar.
8. Pick in the basil.
9. Spoon a layer of tomato sauce into a baking dish.
10. Add a scattering of Parmesan, then single layer of aubergines.
11. Repeat these layers until all the ingredients are used.
12. Toss chopped oregano with breadcrumbs and some olive oil.
13. Sprinkle on top of the Parmesan.
14. Tear over the mozzarella.
15. Let bake 30 minutes.
16. Serve and enjoy.

Bubble and squeak

Ingredients

- 600g of leftover cooked vegetables.
- 600g of leftover roast potatoes
- olive oil
- leftover vac-packed shell nuts
- 25g of unsalted butter
- 4 sprigs of fresh woody herbs

Directions

1. Place a non-stick frying pan on a medium heat with little olive oil and butter.
2. Pick in the fresh herb leaves, let crisp up briefly.
3. Add the potatoes, vegetables, and any leftover shell nuts.
4. Season with sea salt and black pepper.
5. Let cook for 4 minutes or until golden crust forms on the bottom.
6. Using a fish slice, fold crispy bits back into the mash.
7. Let crisp up again, then repeat the process for 20 minutes.
8. Taste and adjust the seasoning accordingly.
9. Serve and enjoy with fried eggs and or lemon-dressed watercress.

Speedy quiche tray bake

Ingredients

- 6 medium free-range eggs
- 1 x 250g pack of ready-rolled filo pastry
- 55g of mature Cheddar cheese
- 1 large courgette
- 1 bunch of spring onions
- Olive oil
- 300g of broccoli

Directions

1. Start by preheating the oven ready to 350°F.
2. Then, grease a large roasting tray with bit of olive oil.
3. Crack the eggs into a bowl and beat well.
4. Layer the filo sheets into the tray, laying one sheet horizontally, and the next vertically, repeating as you layer.
5. Bush with bit of egg between each sheet.
6. Add a final brush to the last layer and scrunch up any excess pastry.
7. Add slice spring onions, cheddar cheese, courgette, and broccoli to the bowl.
8. Season with sea salt and black pepper, mix.

9. Pour the mixture into the prepared pastry case, spreading out.

10. Sprinkle the remaining cheese over the top.

11. Let cook for 35 minutes, until the pastry is golden.

12. Serve and enjoy.

Roasted parsnips

This recipe is infused with the acidity of the vinegar that strikes through the entire recipe with bay and honey.

Ingredients

- 4 fresh bay leaves
- 2 tablespoons of runny honey
- 1.5kg of medium parsnips
- 1 tablespoon of white or red wine vinegar
- 50g of unsalted butter

Directions

1. Firstly, preheat your oven ready to 350°F.
2. Blanch whole in a large pan of boiling salted water for 5 minutes.
3. Drain off the water and steam dry.
4. Tip into a large roasting tray.
5. Dot over the butter and a pinch of sea salt and black pepper, toss to coat.
6. Organize in a single layer, let roast for at least 1 hour.
7. Remove from oven, quickly scatter over the bay leaves.
8. Drizzle with the vinegar and honey, toss together.
9. Continue to roast for 10 minutes or until golden.
10. Serve and enjoy.

Veggie Bolognese sauce

Ingredients

- 250g of alliums
- 1 liter tomato base sauce
- 12g of garlic
- 1 tablespoon of dried mixed herbs
- 1 veggie stock cube
- 750g of Mediterranean veggies
- 25ml of olive oil
- 250g of lentils

Directions

1. Place a large pan to hold all the ingredients on a medium heat with the olive oil.
2. Add the alliums together with the garlic.
3. Let cook for 20 minutes.
4. Add the chopped Mediterranean vegetables with the herbs.
5. Let cook for 15 minutes or until the vegetables are golden.
6. Crush the vegetables.
7. Add the lentils with the tomato base sauce, boil.
8. Add water and stock cube stir well.
9. Boil, lower the heat, let simmer for 40 minutes.
10. Season with sea salt and black pepper.
11. Serve and enjoy.

Veggie korma

Ingredients

- 2 x 400g tins of chickpeas
- 500g of alliums
- lemon juice
- 175g of plain yoghurt
- 350ml of white base sauce
- 30ml of olive oil
- 2 tablespoons of curry powder
- 2 teaspoons of smoked paprika
- 1kg of mixed vegetables
- 750ml of curry base sauce

Directions

1. Place all the ingredients in large a pan over medium heat with the oil.
2. Add the alliums together with the curry powder and smoked paprika.
3. Cook until the alliums are golden in 20 minutes stirring frequently.
4. Add chopped vegetables apart form leafy greens, to the pan, cover let cook briefly.

5. Pour in the curry and white sauces with the chickpeas and water.
6. Bring to the boil, lower the heat let simmer for 35 minutes.
7. Add the reserved leafy vegetables.
8. Boil again, let cook until the curry has reduced.
9. Stir in the yoghurt until warmed through.
10. Season with lemon juice, salt and black pepper.
11. Serve and enjoy.

Freezer raid springtime risotto

Ingredients

- 300g of mixed frozen green vegetables
- 1 liter of vegetable stock
- Extra virgin olive oil
- 1 onion
- 1 stick of celery
- 60g of freshly grated parmesan cheese
- 1 lemon
- Olive oil
- 2 knobs of unsalted butter
- 300g of risotto rice
- 125ml of white wine

Directions

1. Simmer the stock in a pan over a low heat.
2. Place 1 tablespoon of olive oil together with knob of butter, onion, and celery into a pan over low heat.
3. Season lightly with sea salt and black pepper.
4. Cook for 10 minutes, stirring occasionally, until the vegetables are soft.
5. Increase the heat to medium.

6. Add the rice and stir for 2 minutes, pour in the wine and stir to absorb.
7. Add hot stock, stir until fully absorbed, then add more.
8. Cook for 18 minutes, adding more stock every minute, stirring regularly.
9. Stir in the frozen veggies to cook through 5 minutes to rice cook time.
10. Stir in the remaining butter and the Parmesan, season accordingly when heat is off.
11. Drizzle with extra virgin olive oil, squeeze in bit of lemon juice per portion.
12. Enjoy.

Glazed carrots

Ingredients

- 50g of unsalted butter
- 2 fresh bay leaves
- 1 tablespoon of dripping
- 2 clementine
- 2 tablespoons of runny honey
- 1kg of small mixed-color carrots
- 6 cloves of garlic
- 8 sprigs of fresh thyme

Directions

1. Melt the butter in a large frying pan over a medium heat.
2. Add crushed garlic to the pan, turn frequently.
3. Sprinkle in the thyme sprigs, clementine juice and honey, bay, and a splash of water.
4. Add the carrots, sprinkle with sea salt and black pepper, shake to coat.
5. Cover, lower heat to medium-low let cook for 15 minutes.
6. Serve and enjoy.

Brussels sprouts

The Brussels sprouts are insanely delicious with apple cubes, Worcestershire and sausages for a great Mediterranean Sea diet.

Ingredients

- 1 sweet eating apple
- 1 tablespoon of Worcestershire sauce
- 2 higher-welfare Cumberland sausages
- 1 onion
- 800g of Brussels sprouts
- ½ a bunch of fresh sage
- 20g of unsalted butter

Directions

1. Cook the Brussels in a large pan of boiling salted water for 5 minutes.
2. Drain any excess water, let steam dry.
3. Melt butter in a large frying pan on a medium-low heat.
4. Add half the sage leaves and let cook for 3 minutes, transfer into a small bowl.

5. Place the pan back on the heat, add the sausage to the pan.
6. Cook for 5 minutes, until golden.
7. Add the onion with the chopped sage let cook for 5 minutes over medium heat, stirring occasionally.
8. Add sliced apples with sprouts, Worcestershire sauce and toss.
9. Serve and enjoy with scatter sage leaves on top.

Crispy Moroccan carrots

Ingredients

- 6 tablespoons of natural yoghurt
- 12 baby carrots
- Runny honey
- 3 oranges
- 2 teaspoons of rose harissa
- 1 tablespoon of tahini
- 3 fresh bay leaves
- 2 tablespoons of sesame seeds
- 3 sprigs of fresh thyme
- 4 sheets of filo pastry
- Olive oil

Directions

1. Preheat the oven ready to 400°F.
2. Place and cook the carrots in a pan of fast-boiling salted water for 10 minutes.
3. Drain any excess water.
4. Grate half the orange zest into the empty pan with all the juice.
5. Place on a medium heat.

6. Add the bay with thyme and a pinch of sea salt, let cook until syrupy.
7. Fold carrots back into the glaze to coat. Let cool.
8. Lay out the filo sheets rubbed with oil, then cut lengthways into 3 strips.
9. Place a carrot at the bottom of each and roll up.
10. Repeat for all the carrots and filo.
11. Transfer to a baking tray.
12. Brush each lightly with oil, let roast for 20 minutes.
13. Drizzle with a little honey and scattering with the sesame seeds for last 5 minutes.
14. Stack the carrots on a board, swirl the tahini and harissa through the yoghurt.
15. Serve and enjoy.

Rogan josh scotch eggs

Ingredients

- mango chutney
- 5 large free-range eggs
- 2 liters of vegetable oil
- 2 x 250 g packets of mixed cooked grains
- 50g of plain flour
- 2 heaped teaspoons of Rogan josh curry paste
- 1 bunch of fresh mint
- 1 naan bread

Directions

1. Start by soft-boiling 4 eggs in a pan of boiling salted water on a medium heat for 5 minutes.
2. Drain, let cool under running water. Peel.
3. Place the grains into a food processor with the curry paste, mint leaves, process until tacky in texture.
4. Divide into 4 balls.
5. Pat one at a time on a greaseproof paper.
6. Place the paper flat on your hand, put a peeled egg in the center and mold the mixture up and around the egg to seal it inside.

7. Remove the ball from the paper, press in hands to create the perfect covering.

8. Place the flour in one bowl, beat the remaining egg in a separate bowl, add the naan to fine crumbs into a third bowl.

9. Cover the coated eggs with flour, dip into the beaten egg and roll in the crumbs.

10. Place on a medium-high heat.

11. Lower the Scotch eggs into the pan let cook for 8 minutes.

12. Scoop out and drain on kitchen paper.

13. Serve and enjoy.

Cherry clafoutis

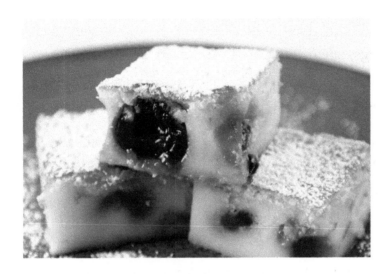

Ingredients

- 60g of sugar
- ½ tablespoon of unsalted butter
- 1 tablespoon of sugar
- ½ teaspoon of vanilla extract
- 300g of cherries
- 300ml of milk
- Icing sugar
- ½ teaspoon of baking powder
- 3 large free-range eggs
- 60g of plain flour

Directions

1. Preheat the oven to 360°F.

2. Combine plain four together with the baking powder, eggs, sugar, milk, and vanilla extract in a food processor, blend until smooth, keep for 30 minutes.

3. Oil a round baking dish with the softened butter.

4. Sprinkle over with the sugar.

5. Dot the cherries around the base, place in the oven for 5 minutes.

6. Remove and pour over the batter until the cherries are just covered.

7. Return to the oven let bake for 35 minutes.

8. Dust the clafoutis with icing sugar and serve warm.

9. Enjoy.

Cranberry Bakewell

Ingredients

- 2 large eggs
- 375g of sweet short crust pastry
- 2 heaped tablespoons of plain flour
- 1 splash calvados
- 1 handful of cranberries, fresh, defrosted
- 250g of unsalted butter
- 1 orange
- 100g of icing sugar
- 375g of cranberries, fresh or defrosted
- 150g of golden caster sugar
- 1-star anise
- 1 orange
- 1/2 teaspoon of ground cinnamon
- 1 vanilla pod
- 300g of ground almonds
- 300g of golden caster sugar

Directions

1. Grate the orange zest into a pan.
2. Squeeze in the juice, let simmer with the remaining ingredients, stirring occasionally.

3. Taste, and adjust accordingly.

4. Cool, then remove the star anise.

5. Roll out the pastry to line oiled loose-bottomed tart tin.

6. Let chill in the fridge for 1 hour.

7. Combine vanilla pod, almonds, plain flour, caster sugar, eggs, unsalted butter, and processor, process until smooth.

8. Wrap in Clingfilm and chill in the fridge for 30 minutes with pastry.

9. Preheat the oven ready to 380°F.

10. Line the pastry with greaseproof paper and fill with dried beans.

11. Let bake for 10 minutes.

12. Remove the beans and paper continue to bake for more 15 minutes.

13. Remove.

14. Then, spread the pastry with the jam, dollop over the frangipane.

15. Sprinkle with the cranberries, scatter with flaked almonds.

16. Bake 55 minutes.

17. Let tart cool.

18. Grate the orange zest into a small bowl.

19. Add the icing sugar, squeeze enough orange juice to give a drizzling consistency.

20. Serve and enjoy with crème fraiche.

Winter ginger, pear and almond cake

The winter ginger, pear and almond recipe is known for its aromatic ginger flavor with spicy sweet satisfying ingredients.

It is an incredible Mediterranean Sea fruit recipe for a perfect breakfast choice.

Ingredients

- 20g of butter
- 220g of ground almonds
- 300g of ginger
- 4 pears
- 200g of butter
- 1 vanilla pod
- 200g of caster sugar
- 550g of caster sugar
- 4 large free-range eggs

Directions

1. Preheat the oven ready to 380°F.
2. Place the vanilla pod, grated ginger, and pears into a pan.

3. Add 400g sugar and water let boil, simmer for briefly.

4. Lower the pears into the hot liquid, simmer for 10 minutes.

5. Remove the pears from the liquid let cool.

6. Line a cake tin with greaseproof paper.

7. Combine the remaining 150g sugar and water in a pan over a high heat.

8. Simmer for 15 minutes until dark golden brown.

9. Stir in the butter until you get a caramel, then pour into cake tin.

10. Slices cooled pears, arrange in the warm caramel.

11. Mix butter with sugar until smooth.

12. Add the eggs one at a time, mix well one after the other.

13. Add the almonds and mix to combine.

14. Pour the cake mixture over the pears let bake 35 minutes in the heated oven.

15. Serve and enjoy.

Summer pudding

Ingredients

- 2 tablespoons of red berry jam
- 150g of sugar
- ½ of an orange
- ½ teaspoon of vanilla paste
- 800g of mixed summer berries
- Olive oil
- 7 large slices of white bread

Directions

1. Grease a pudding basin with oil.
2. Align with 2 sheets of Clingfilm.
3. Place the berries in a large saucepan together with the sugar, orange juice, and vanilla paste.
4. Over low heat, let cook for 5 minutes or till the juices start bleeding from the fruit. Let cool.
5. Remove the crusts from the bread, spread over the jam.
6. Line the basin with 6 of the slices, jam-side up with no gaps.
7. Press the bread against the sides.
8. Spoon the cooled fruit and pour its juice into the lined basin, reserving some.

9. Cover the pudding with the last slice of bread, jam-side down.

10. Place a saucer that fits inside the basin on top of the pudding, then place a weight, on top.

11. Refrigerate 12 hours to soak the juices.

12. Strain the leftover juice through a fine sieve into a small pan.

13. Let boil, simmer for 10 minutes.

14. Drizzle large slices with the syrup.

15. Serve and enjoy with crème fraiche.

Raspberry burnt cream

Ingredients

- 100g of raspberries
- 150ml of double cream
- 4 large free-range egg yolks
- 1 vanilla pod
- 2 tablespoons of golden caster sugar
- 150ml of single cream

Directions

1. Preheat the oven to 300°F.
2. Add vanilla pod to a pan with the creams over a low heat.
3. In a bowl, whisk the egg yolks with sugar.
4. Add in the hot cream, whisk frequently to make a custard.
5. Strain through a sieve into a jug.
6. Boil water.
7. Divide the berries between four small ovenproof ramekins, then fill each with the custard.
8. Place ramekins in roasting tray, pour in hot water halfway up the sides.
9. Let cook in the oven for 20 minutes.
10. Remove, let cool, then cover each ramekin with Clingfilm, refrigerate overnight.

11. Sprinkle sugar over the custards, burn the top with a blowtorch.
12. Allow to stand to let the burnt sugar hardens, then return to the fridge and chill until needed.
13. Enjoy.

Citrus poached pears

Ingredients

- Double cream
- 1 lemon
- 2 pears
- 1 stick of cinnamon
- 200g of granulated sugar
- 1 orange

Directions

1. Place the peeled zest and juice from the lemon, orange into a saucepan.
2. Add the cinnamon together with the sugar, add 500ml of water and bring to the boil, until the sugar dissolves.
3. Add the pears into the syrup once the sugar has dissolved.
4. Let simmer 12 minutes or until tender.
5. Remove and let cool.
6. Serve the pears with double cream and or with 4 tablespoons of poaching.
7. Enjoy.

Limon cello and fruit salad fro-yo

Ingredients

- 75ml of Limon cello
- 1kg of chopped mixed fruit
- Ice-cream cones
- 250ml of fat-free natural yoghurt
- Runny honey

Directions

1. Blend the fruit together with the yoghurt, 2 tablespoons of honey, and the limon cello in a food processor until smooth.
2. Taste and adjust accordingly.
3. Spoon into a dish and freeze for 2 hours, until frozen.
4. Remove and place back into the processor, blend again to break up any ice crystals. Enjoy.

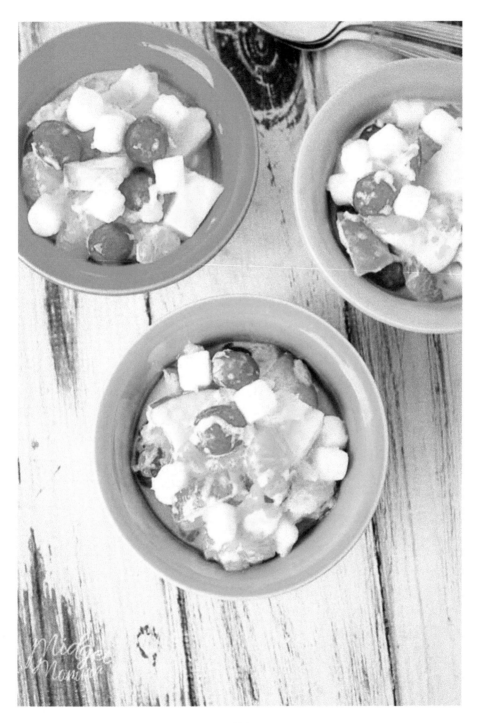